Self Care Isn't Selfish

A Guided Journal to Express Yourself and Really Practice Self Care

Self Care Isn't Selfish

Dedication

I dedicate this book to everyone who has ever pushed themselves way too much and needed a break. Thank you for supporting.

Love,

-LaShonda Bracey

Introduction

I created this journal to do be used as a guide for self care we are often consumed with taking care of everyone else that we often neglect ourselves.

This journal is meant to be used daily as a way to take a step back and relax?

-LaShonda Bracey

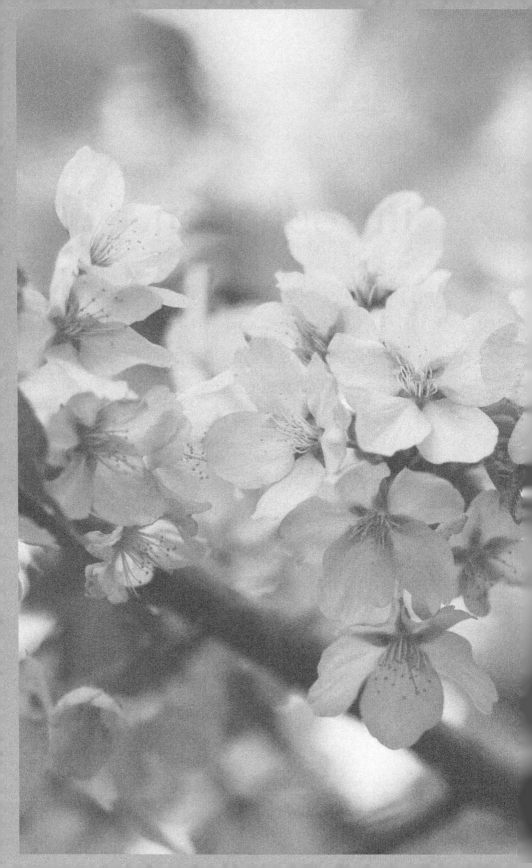

Daily Self-Care
Q&A

How do I feel today?

_____

What I am thankful for right now?

_____

What negative attitude do I need to change?

_____

What positive affirmation was I able to
give myself today?

_____

What ongoing support do I need?

_____

What do I need to do to be a better version of myself?

_____

Daily Self-Care Q&A

How do I feel today?

_____

What I am thankful for right now?

_____

What negative attitude do I need to change?

_____

What positive affirmation was I able to give myself today?

_____

What ongoing support do I need?

_____

What do I need to do to be a better version of myself?

_____

Daily Self-Care
Q&A

How do I feel today?

_____

What I am thankful for right now?

_____

What negative attitude do I need to change?

_____

What positive affirmation was I able to
give myself today?

_____

What ongoing support do I need?

_____

What do I need to do to be a better version of myself?

_____

Daily Self-Care Q&A

How do I feel today?

_____

What I am thankful for right now?

_____

What negative attitude do I need to change?

_____

What positive affirmation was I able to
give myself today?

_____

What ongoing support do I need?

_____

What do I need to do to be a better version of myself?

_____

Daily Self-Care
Q&A

How do I feel today?

_____

What I am thankful for right now?

_____

What negative attitude do I need to change?

_____

What positive affirmation was I able to
give myself today?

_____

What ongoing support do I need?

_____

What do I need to do to be a better version of myself?

_____

Daily Self-Care Q&A

How do I feel today?

_____

What I am thankful for right now?

_____

What negative attitude do I need to change?

_____

What positive affirmation was I able to
give myself today?

_____

What ongoing support do I need?

_____

What do I need to do to be a better version of myself?

_____

Daily Self-Care
Q&A

Date:_____

How do I feel today?

_____

What I am thankful for right now?

_____

What negative attitude do I need to change?

_____

What positive affirmation was I able to
give myself today?

_____

What ongoing support do I need?

_____

What do I need to do to be a better version of myself?

_____

Daily Self-Care Q&A

How do I feel today?

_____

What I am thankful for right now?

_____

What negative attitude do I need to change?

_____

What positive affirmation was I able to
give myself today?

_____

What ongoing support do I need?

_____

What do I need to do to be a better version of myself?

_____

Daily Self-Care
Q&A

How do I feel today?

_____

What I am thankful for right now?

_____

What negative attitude do I need to change?

_____

What positive affirmation was I able to
give myself today?

_____

What ongoing support do I need?

_____

What do I need to do to be a better version of myself?

_____

Daily Self-Care Q&A

ANSWER HONESTLY!   Date:_____

How do I feel today?

_____

What I am thankful for right now?

_____

What negative attitude do I need to change?

_____

What positive affirmation was I able to give myself today?

_____

What ongoing support do I need?

_____

What do I need to do to be a better version of myself?

_____

Daily Self-Care Q&A

How do I feel today?

_____

What I am thankful for right now?

_____

What negative attitude do I need to change?

_____

What positive affirmation was I able to
give myself today?

_____

What ongoing support do I need?

_____

What do I need to do to be a better version of myself?

_____

Daily Self-Care Q&A

How do I feel today?

_____

What I am thankful for right now?

_____

What negative attitude do I need to change?

_____

What positive affirmation was I able to
give myself today?

_____

What ongoing support do I need?

_____

What do I need to do to be a better version of myself?

_____

Daily Self-Care
Q&A

Date:_____

How do I feel today?

_____

What I am thankful for right now?

_____

What negative attitude do I need to change?

_____

What positive affirmation was I able to
give myself today?

_____

What ongoing support do I need?

_____

What do I need to do to be a better version of myself?

_____

Daily Self-Care Q&A

How do I feel today?

_____

What I am thankful for right now?

_____

What negative attitude do I need to change?

_____

What positive affirmation was I able to
give myself today?

_____

What ongoing support do I need?

_____

What do I need to do to be a better version of myself?

_____

Daily Self-Care Q&A

How do I feel today?

_____

What I am thankful for right now?

_____

What negative attitude do I need to change?

_____

What positive affirmation was I able to
give myself today?

_____

What ongoing support do I need?

_____

What do I need to do to be a better version of myself?

_____

Daily Self-Care
Q&A

How do I feel today?

_____

What I am thankful for right now?

_____

What negative attitude do I need to change?

_____

What positive affirmation was I able to
give myself today?

_____

What ongoing support do I need?

_____

What do I need to do to be a better version of myself?

_____

Daily Self-Care
Q&A

How do I feel today?

_____

What I am thankful for right now?

_____

What negative attitude do I need to change?

_____

_____

What positive affirmation was I able to
give myself today?
What ongoing support do I need?

_____

What do I need to do to be a better version of myself?

_____

Daily Self-Care Q&A

How do I feel today?

_____

What I am thankful for right now?

_____

What negative attitude do I need to change?

_____

What positive affirmation was I able to
give myself today?

_____

What ongoing support do I need?

_____

What do I need to do to be a better version of myself?

_____

Daily Self-Care
Q&A

Date:_____

How do I feel today?

_____

What I am thankful for right now?

_____

What negative attitude do I need to change?

_____

What positive affirmation was I able to
give myself today?

_____

What ongoing support do I need?

_____

What do I need to do to be a better version of myself?

_____

Daily Self-Care Q&A

How do I feel today?

_____

What I am thankful for right now?

_____

What negative attitude do I need to change?

_____

What positive affirmation was I able to
give myself today?

_____

What ongoing support do I need?

_____

What do I need to do to be a better version of myself?

_____

Daily Self-Care
Q&A

How do I feel today?

_____

What I am thankful for right now?

_____

What negative attitude do I need to change?

_____

What positive affirmation was I able to
give myself today?

_____

What ongoing support do I need?

_____

What do I need to do to be a better version of myself?

_____

Daily Self-Care Q&A

ANSWER HONESTLY!   Date:_____

How do I feel today?

_____

What I am thankful for right now?

_____

What negative attitude do I need to change?

_____

What positive affirmation was I able to
give myself today?

_____

What ongoing support do I need?

_____

What do I need to do to be a better version of myself?

_____

Daily Self-Care Q&A

ANSWER HONESTLY!   Date:_____

How do I feel today?

_____

What I am thankful for right now?

_____

What negative attitude do I need to change?

_____

What positive affirmation was I able to
give myself today?

_____

What ongoing support do I need?

_____

What do I need to do to be a better version of myself?

_____

Daily Self-Care Q&A

ANSWER HONESTLY!   Date:_____

How do I feel today?

_____

What I am thankful for right now?

_____

What negative attitude do I need to change?

_____

What positive affirmation was I able to
give myself today?

_____

What ongoing support do I need?

_____

What do I need to do to be a better version of myself?

_____

Daily Self-Care Q&A

How do I feel today?

_____

What I am thankful for right now?

_____

What negative attitude do I need to change?

_____

What positive affirmation was I able to
give myself today?

_____

What ongoing support do I need?

_____

What do I need to do to be a better version of myself?

_____

Daily Self-Care Q&A

How do I feel today?

_____

What I am thankful for right now?

_____

What negative attitude do I need to change?

_____

What positive affirmation was I able to
give myself today?

_____

What ongoing support do I need?

_____

What do I need to do to be a better version of myself?

_____

Daily Self-Care Q&A

How do I feel today?

_____

What I am thankful for right now?

_____

What negative attitude do I need to change?

_____

What positive affirmation was I able to
give myself today?

_____

What ongoing support do I need?

_____

What do I need to do to be a better version of myself?

_____

Daily Self-Care Q&A

How do I feel today?

_____

What I am thankful for right now?

_____

What negative attitude do I need to change?

_____

What positive affirmation was I able to
give myself today?

_____

What ongoing support do I need?

_____

What do I need to do to be a better version of myself?

_____

Daily Self-Care
Q&A

How do I feel today?

_____

What I am thankful for right now?

_____

What negative attitude do I need to change?

_____

What positive affirmation was I able to
give myself today?

_____

What ongoing support do I need?

_____

What do I need to do to be a better version of myself?

_____

Daily Self-Care Q&A

How do I feel today?

_____

What I am thankful for right now?

_____

What negative attitude do I need to change?

_____

What positive affirmation was I able to
give myself today?

_____

What ongoing support do I need?

_____

What do I need to do to be a better version of myself?

_____

Daily Self-Care Q&A

How do I feel today?

_____

What I am thankful for right now?

_____

What negative attitude do I need to change?

_____

What positive affirmation was I able to
give myself today?

_____

What ongoing support do I need?

_____

What do I need to do to be a better version of myself?

_____

Daily Self-Care Q&A

How do I feel today?

_____

What I am thankful for right now?

_____

What negative attitude do I need to change?

_____

What positive affirmation was I able to give myself today?

_____

What ongoing support do I need?

_____

What do I need to do to be a better version of myself?

_____

Daily Self-Care
Q&A

Date:_____

How do I feel today?

_____

What I am thankful for right now?

_____

What negative attitude do I need to change?

_____

What positive affirmation was I able to
give myself today?

_____

What ongoing support do I need?

_____

What do I need to do to be a better version of myself?

_____

Daily Self-Care
Q&A

How do I feel today?

_____

What I am thankful for right now?

_____

What negative attitude do I need to change?

_____

What positive affirmation was I able to
give myself today?

_____

What ongoing support do I need?

_____

What do I need to do to be a better version of myself?

_____

Daily Self-Care Q&A

Date:_____

How do I feel today?

_____

What I am thankful for right now?

_____

What negative attitude do I need to change?

_____

What positive affirmation was I able to
give myself today?

_____

What ongoing support do I need?

_____

What do I need to do to be a better version of myself?

_____

Daily Self-Care Q&A

How do I feel today?

_____

What I am thankful for right now?

_____

What negative attitude do I need to change?

_____

What positive affirmation was I able to
give myself today?

_____

What ongoing support do I need?

_____

What do I need to do to be a better version of myself?

_____

Daily Self-Care Q&A

How do I feel today?

_____

What I am thankful for right now?

_____

What negative attitude do I need to change?

_____

What positive affirmation was I able to
give myself today?

_____

What ongoing support do I need?

_____

What do I need to do to be a better version of myself?

_____

Daily Self-Care Q&A

Date:_____

How do I feel today?

_____

What I am thankful for right now?

_____

What negative attitude do I need to change?

_____

What positive affirmation was I able to give myself today?

_____

What ongoing support do I need?

_____

What do I need to do to be a better version of myself?

_____

Daily Self-Care
Q&A

How do I feel today?

_____

What I am thankful for right now?

_____

What negative attitude do I need to change?

_____

What positive affirmation was I able to
give myself today?

_____

What ongoing support do I need?

_____

What do I need to do to be a better version of myself?

_____

Daily Self-Care
Q&A

How do I feel today?

_____

What I am thankful for right now?

_____

What negative attitude do I need to change?

_____

What positive affirmation was I able to
give myself today?

_____

What ongoing support do I need?

_____

What do I need to do to be a better version of myself?

_____

Daily Self-Care Q&A

Date:_____

How do I feel today?

_____

What I am thankful for right now?

_____

What negative attitude do I need to change?

_____

What positive affirmation was I able to
give myself today?

_____

What ongoing support do I need?

_____

What do I need to do to be a better version of myself?

_____

Daily Self-Care Q&A

How do I feel today?

_____

What I am thankful for right now?

_____

What negative attitude do I need to change?

_____

What positive affirmation was I able to
give myself today?

_____

What ongoing support do I need?

_____

What do I need to do to be a better version of myself?

_____

Daily Self-Care Q&A

How do I feel today?

_____

What I am thankful for right now?

_____

What negative attitude do I need to change?

_____

What positive affirmation was I able to
give myself today?

_____

What ongoing support do I need?

_____

What do I need to do to be a better version of myself?

_____

Daily Self-Care Q&A

How do I feel today?

_____

What I am thankful for right now?

_____

What negative attitude do I need to change?

_____

What positive affirmation was I able to
give myself today?

_____

What ongoing support do I need?

_____

What do I need to do to be a better version of myself?

_____

Daily Self-Care Q&A

Date:_____

How do I feel today?

_____

What I am thankful for right now?

_____

What negative attitude do I need to change?

_____

What positive affirmation was I able to
give myself today?

_____

What ongoing support do I need?

_____

What do I need to do to be a better version of myself?

_____

Daily Self-Care
Q&A

How do I feel today?

_____

What I am thankful for right now?

_____

What negative attitude do I need to change?

_____

What positive affirmation was I able to
give myself today?

_____

What ongoing support do I need?

_____

What do I need to do to be a better version of myself?

_____

Daily Self-Care
Q&A

How do I feel today?

_____

What I am thankful for right now?

_____

What negative attitude do I need to change?

_____

What positive affirmation was I able to
give myself today?

_____

What ongoing support do I need?

_____

What do I need to do to be a better version of myself?

_____

Daily Self-Care Q&A

How do I feel today?

_____

What I am thankful for right now?

_____

What negative attitude do I need to change?

_____

What positive affirmation was I able to
give myself today?

_____

What ongoing support do I need?

_____

What do I need to do to be a better version of myself?

_____

Daily Self-Care Q&A

How do I feel today?

_____

What I am thankful for right now?

_____

What negative attitude do I need to change?

_____

What positive affirmation was I able to
give myself today?

_____

What ongoing support do I need?

_____

What do I need to do to be a better version of myself?

_____

Daily Self-Care
Q&A

How do I feel today?

_____

What I am thankful for right now?

_____

What negative attitude do I need to change?

_____

What positive affirmation was I able to
give myself today?

_____

What ongoing support do I need?

_____

What do I need to do to be a better version of myself?

_____

Daily Self-Care Q&A

How do I feel today?

_____

What I am thankful for right now?

_____

What negative attitude do I need to change?

_____

What positive affirmation was I able to
give myself today?

_____

What ongoing support do I need?

_____

What do I need to do to be a better version of myself?

_____

Daily Self-Care
Q&A

ANSWER HONESTLY!　　　　　Date:_____

How do I feel today?

_____

What I am thankful for right now?

_____

What negative attitude do I need to change?

_____

What positive affirmation was I able to
give myself today?

_____

What ongoing support do I need?

_____

What do I need to do to be a better version of myself?

_____

Daily Self-Care Q&A

How do I feel today?

_____

What I am thankful for right now?

_____

What negative attitude do I need to change?

_____

What positive affirmation was I able to
give myself today?

_____

What ongoing support do I need?

_____

What do I need to do to be a better version of myself?

_____

Daily Self-Care Q&A

How do I feel today?

_____

What I am thankful for right now?

_____

What negative attitude do I need to change?

_____

What positive affirmation was I able to
give myself today?

_____

What ongoing support do I need?

_____

What do I need to do to be a better version of myself?

_____

Daily Self-Care
Q&A

How do I feel today?

_____

What I am thankful for right now?

_____

What negative attitude do I need to change?

_____

What positive affirmation was I able to
give myself today?

_____

What ongoing support do I need?

_____

What do I need to do to be a better version of myself?

_____

Daily Self-Care
Q&A

How do I feel today?

_____

What I am thankful for right now?

_____

What negative attitude do I need to change?

_____

What positive affirmation was I able to
give myself today?

_____

What ongoing support do I need?

_____

What do I need to do to be a better version of myself?

_____

Daily Self-Care
Q&A

How do I feel today?

_____

What I am thankful for right now?

_____

What negative attitude do I need to change?

_____

What positive affirmation was I able to
give myself today?

_____

What ongoing support do I need?

_____

Daily Self-Care Q&A

ANSWER HONESTLY!   Date:_____

How do I feel today?

_____

What I am thankful for right now?

_____

What negative attitude do I need to change?

_____

What positive affirmation was I able to
give myself today?

_____

What ongoing support do I need?

_____

What do I need to do to be a better version of myself?

_____

Daily Self-Care
Q&A

Date:_____

How do I feel today?

_____

What I am thankful for right now?

_____

What negative attitude do I need to change?

_____

What positive affirmation was I able to
give myself today?

_____

What ongoing support do I need?

_____

What do I need to do to be a better version of myself?

_____

Daily Self-Care Q&A

How do I feel today?

_____

What I am thankful for right now?

_____

What negative attitude do I need to change?

_____

_____

What ongoing support do I need?

_____

What do I need to do to be a better version of myself?

_____

Daily Self-Care Q&A

How do I feel today?

_____

What I am thankful for right now?

_____

What negative attitude do I need to change?

_____

What positive affirmation was I able to
give myself today?

_____

What ongoing support do I need?

_____

What do I need to do to be a better version of myself?

_____

Daily Self-Care Q&A

How do I feel today?

_____

What I am thankful for right now?

_____

What negative attitude do I need to change?

_____

What positive affirmation was I able to give myself today?

_____

What ongoing support do I need?

_____

What do I need to do to be a better version of myself?

_____

Daily Self-Care Q&A

How do I feel today?

_____

What I am thankful for right now?

_____

What negative attitude do I need to change?

_____

What positive affirmation was I able to
give myself today?

_____

What ongoing support do I need?

_____

What do I need to do to be a better version of myself?

_____

Daily Self-Care Q&A

Date:_____

How do I feel today?

_____

What I am thankful for right now?

_____

What negative attitude do I need to change?

_____

What positive affirmation was I able to
give myself today?

_____

What ongoing support do I need?

_____

What do I need to do to be a better version of myself?

_____

Daily Self-Care
Q&A

How do I feel today?

_____

What I am thankful for right now?

_____

What negative attitude do I need to change?

_____

What positive affirmation was I able to
give myself today?

_____

What ongoing support do I need?

_____

What do I need to do to be a better version of myself?

_____

Daily Self-Care Q&A

How do I feel today?

_____

What I am thankful for right now?

_____

What negative attitude do I need to change?

_____

What positive affirmation was I able to
give myself today?

_____

What ongoing support do I need?

_____

What do I need to do to be a better version of myself?

_____

Daily Self-Care
Q&A

ANSWER HONESTLY!   Date:_____

How do I feel today?

_____

What I am thankful for right now?

_____

What negative attitude do I need to change?

_____

What positive affirmation was I able to
give myself today?

_____

What ongoing support do I need?

_____

What do I need to do to be a better version of myself?

_____

Daily Self-Care
Q&A

Date:_____

How do I feel today?

_____

What I am thankful for right now?

_____

What negative attitude do I need to change?

_____

What positive affirmation was I able to
give myself today?

_____

What ongoing support do I need?

_____

What do I need to do to be a better version of myself?

_____

Daily Self-Care
Q&A

How do I feel today?

_____

What I am thankful for right now?

_____

What negative attitude do I need to change?

_____

What positive affirmation was I able to
give myself today?

_____

What ongoing support do I need?

_____

What do I need to do to be a better version of myself?

_____

Daily Self-Care
Q&A

Date:_____

How do I feel today?

_____

What I am thankful for right now?

_____

What negative attitude do I need to change?

_____

What positive affirmation was I able to
give myself today?

_____

What ongoing support do I need?

_____

What do I need to do to be a better version of myself?

_____

Daily Self-Care Q&A

Date:_____

How do I feel today?

_____

What I am thankful for right now?

_____

What negative attitude do I need to change?

_____

What positive affirmation was I able to
give myself today?

_____

What ongoing support do I need?

_____

What do I need to do to be a better version of myself?

_____

Daily Self-Care Q&A

How do I feel today?

_____

What I am thankful for right now?

_____

What negative attitude do I need to change?

_____

What positive affirmation was I able to
give myself today?

_____

What ongoing support do I need?

_____

What do I need to do to be a better version of myself?

_____

Daily Self-Care Q&A

How do I feel today?

_____

What I am thankful for right now?

_____

What negative attitude do I need to change?

_____

What positive affirmation was I able to
give myself today?

_____

What ongoing support do I need?

_____

What do I need to do to be a better version of myself?

_____

Daily Self-Care Q&A

How do I feel today?

_____

What I am thankful for right now?

_____

What negative attitude do I need to change?

_____

What positive affirmation was I able to
give myself today?

_____

What ongoing support do I need?

_____

What do I need to do to be a better version of myself?

_____

Daily Self-Care
Q&A

How do I feel today?

_____

What I am thankful for right now?

_____

What negative attitude do I need to change?

_____

What positive affirmation was I able to
give myself today?

_____

What ongoing support do I need?

_____

What do I need to do to be a better version of myself?

_____

Daily Self-Care Q&A

How do I feel today?

_____

What I am thankful for right now?

_____

What negative attitude do I need to change?

_____

What positive affirmation was I able to
give myself today?

_____

What ongoing support do I need?

_____

What do I need to do to be a better version of myself?

_____

Daily Self-Care
Q&A

How do I feel today?

_____

What I am thankful for right now?

_____

What negative attitude do I need to change?

_____

What positive affirmation was I able to
give myself today?

_____

What ongoing support do I need?

_____

What do I need to do to be a better version of myself?

_____

Daily Self-Care Q&A

How do I feel today?

_____

What I am thankful for right now?

_____

What negative attitude do I need to change?

_____

What positive affirmation was I able to
give myself today?

_____

What ongoing support do I need?

_____

What do I need to do to be a better version of myself?

_____

Daily Self-Care
Q&A

How do I feel today?

_____

What I am thankful for right now?

_____

What negative attitude do I need to change?

_____

What positive affirmation was I able to
give myself today?

_____

What ongoing support do I need?

_____

What do I need to do to be a better version of myself?

_____

Daily Self-Care Q&A

ANSWER HONESTLY!   Date:_____

How do I feel today?

_____

What I am thankful for right now?

_____

What negative attitude do I need to change?

_____

What positive affirmation was I able to
give myself today?

_____

What ongoing support do I need?

_____

What do I need to do to be a better version of myself?

_____

Daily Self-Care
Q&A

How do I feel today?

_____

What I am thankful for right now?

_____

What negative attitude do I need to change?

_____

What positive affirmation was I able to
give myself today?

_____

What ongoing support do I need?

_____

What do I need to do to be a better version of myself?

_____

Daily Self-Care Q&A

Date:_____

How do I feel today?

_____

What I am thankful for right now?

_____

What negative attitude do I need to change?

_____

What positive affirmation was I able to
give myself today?

_____

What ongoing support do I need?

_____

What do I need to do to be a better version of myself?

_____

Daily Self-Care Q&A

How do I feel today?

_____

What I am thankful for right now?

_____

What negative attitude do I need to change?

_____

What positive affirmation was I able to
give myself today?

_____

What ongoing support do I need?

_____

What do I need to do to be a better version of myself?

_____

Daily Self-Care Q&A

How do I feel today?

_____

What I am thankful for right now?

_____

What negative attitude do I need to change?

_____

What positive affirmation was I able to
give myself today?

_____

What ongoing support do I need?

_____

What do I need to do to be a better version of myself?

_____

Daily Self-Care
Q&A

How do I feel today?

_____

What I am thankful for right now?

_____

What negative attitude do I need to change?

_____

What positive affirmation was I able to
give myself today?

_____

What ongoing support do I need?

_____

What do I need to do to be a better version of myself?

_____

Daily Self-Care Q&A

Date:_____

How do I feel today?

_____

What I am thankful for right now?

_____

What negative attitude do I need to change?

_____

What positive affirmation was I able to
give myself today?

_____

What ongoing support do I need?

_____

What do I need to do to be a better version of myself?

_____

Daily Self-Care Q&A

How do I feel today?

_____

What I am thankful for right now?

_____

What negative attitude do I need to change?

_____

What positive affirmation was I able to
give myself today?

_____

What ongoing support do I need?

_____

What do I need to do to be a better version of myself?

_____

Daily Self-Care
Q&A

ANSWER HONESTLY!   Date:_____

How do I feel today?

_____

What I am thankful for right now?

_____

What negative attitude do I need to change?

_____

What positive affirmation was I able to
give myself today?

_____

What ongoing support do I need?

_____

What do I need to do to be a better version of myself?

_____

Daily Self-Care
Q&A

How do I feel today?

_____

What I am thankful for right now?

_____

What negative attitude do I need to change?

_____

What positive affirmation was I able to
give myself today?

_____

What ongoing support do I need?

_____

What do I need to do to be a better version of myself?

_____

Daily Self-Care Q&A

How do I feel today?

_____

What I am thankful for right now?

_____

What negative attitude do I need to change?

_____

What positive affirmation was I able to
give myself today?

_____

What ongoing support do I need?

_____

What do I need to do to be a better version of myself?

_____

Daily Self-Care
Q&A

Date:_____

How do I feel today?

_____

What I am thankful for right now?

_____

What negative attitude do I need to change?

_____

What positive affirmation was I able to
give myself today?

_____

What ongoing support do I need?

_____

What do I need to do to be a better version of myself?

_____

Daily Self-Care Q&A

ANSWER HONESTLY!   Date:_____

How do I feel today?

_____

What I am thankful for right now?

_____

What negative attitude do I need to change?

_____

What positive affirmation was I able to
give myself today?

_____

What ongoing support do I need?

_____

What do I need to do to be a better version of myself?

_____

Daily Self-Care
Q&A

How do I feel today?

_____

What I am thankful for right now?

_____

What negative attitude do I need to change?

_____

What positive affirmation was I able to
give myself today?

_____

What ongoing support do I need?

_____

What do I need to do to be a better version of myself?

_____

Daily Self-Care Q&A

Date:_____

How do I feel today?

_____

What I am thankful for right now?

_____

What negative attitude do I need to change?

_____

What positive affirmation was I able to
give myself today?

_____

What ongoing support do I need?

_____

What do I need to do to be a better version of myself?

_____

Made in the USA
Coppell, TX
22 February 2021